My Cancer Journey

and the

Faith

that sustained me

NAOMI WHITE

NAOMI WHITE

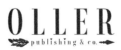
OLLER
publishing & co.

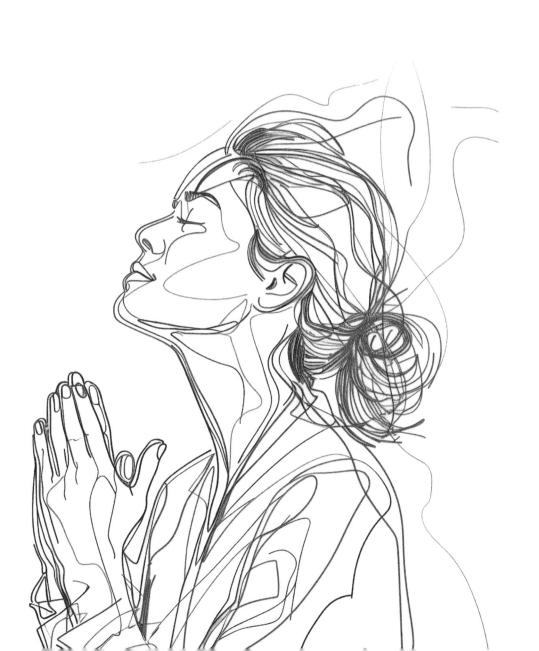

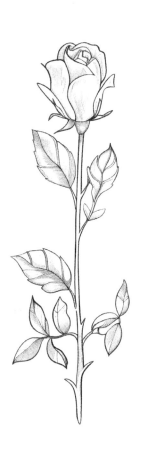

Dedication

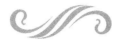

To my two daughters, Nancy, and Kristy, for their tireless dedication to my health and well-being.

And to my mom and dad, for their ceaseless prayers on my behalf.

I couldn't have done it without all of you. All the trips to visit me, all the time spent waiting with me in doctor's offices and chemotherapy sessions, and all the prayers and support that you showed me made this a bearable journey.

I will forever be thankful and grateful for your love and support.

"OCSRI has an unrelenting dedication to patients and families. They are the kindest and most caring people you could ever wish for in your cancer journey. Dr. Gold and Melissa P took such good care of me. I trust them with my life."

Naomi
OCSRI Patient

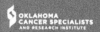

Special Thanks

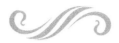

To Dr. Michael Gold and the entire staff at OCSRI for their exceptional dedication to their patients' quality of life and their exemplary level of compassionate care in my hour of need.

You truly are a beacon of light in the darkness, which is cancer. Thank you from the very bottom of my heart.

"OCSRI has an unrelenting dedication to their patients and families. They are the kindest and most caring people you could ever wish for in your cancer journey. I trust them with my life."
-Naomi, OCSRI patient

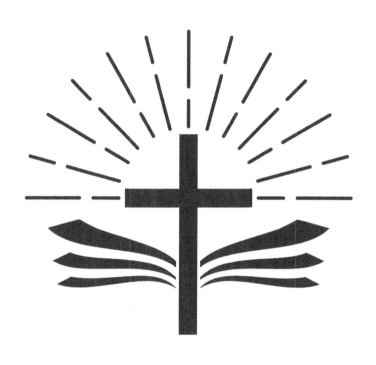

TABLE OF CONTENTS

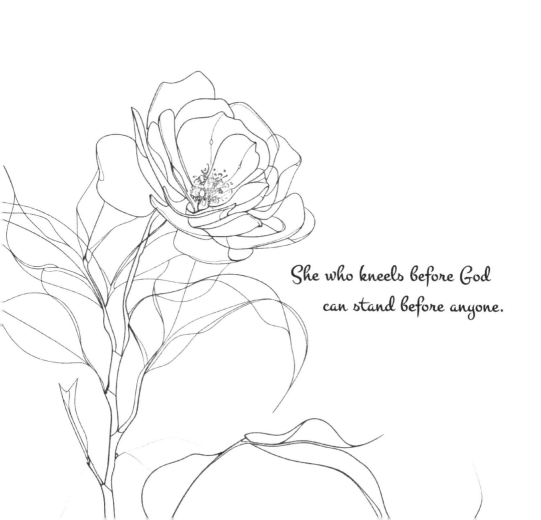

She who kneels before God
can stand before anyone.

Preface

I never expected to be face-to-face with cancer. This is the story of how that came to be for me and how my faith sustained me in the battle for my life. It is a story of Hope and the Power of Prayer. I wrote this as a testament to that power and as an inspiration to you in your own faith journey.

Be strong and courageous. Do not be terrified. Do not be discouraged. For the Lord your God will be with you wherever you go. Joshua 1:9

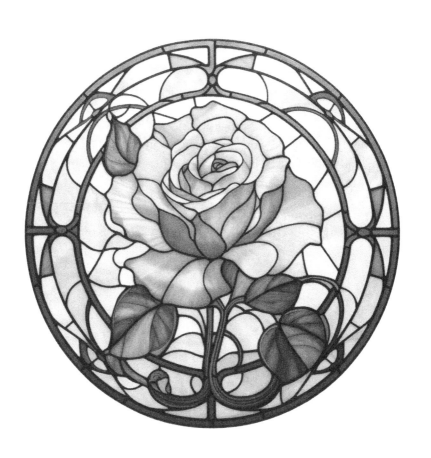

Cancer

That word had always brought to mind kaleidoscopic whirlwinds of incomplete impressions, of lives distorted as if seen through swirling bits of broken colored glass. I'd known friends and acquaintances, even family, who had been on this journey, but I had never been intimately affected by the ever-changing struggles of this disease.

All that was about to change.

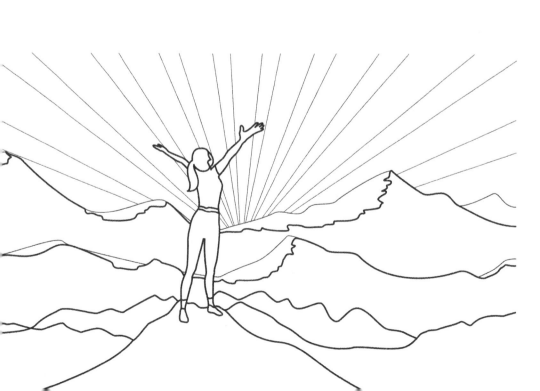

The Beginning

My faith grew firm and unshakable,

a sustaining bedrock for my life.

My faith journey began when I was young. I was raised in a Christian home; my parents both loved God and daily demonstrated their own faith so convincingly that at the age of ten, I, too, proclaimed my faith and accepted my personal call to follow God. I walked down the aisle at a New Year's Eve watch-night service; I was starting my new year with a new life. The faith I embraced from this early age formed a rock-solid foundation that supported and sustained me throughout the rest of my life; this was the beginning of my lifelong journey of faith.

My father was a chaplain in the military, and we moved frequently, often clear across or even out of the country. Our close-knit family did not live near our other relatives, but we were usually able to visit them between moves. I loved the adventures and ever-changing scenery we encountered and grew to love these travels. Because we lived in so many different locations, I learned how to adapt quickly to changing situations and overcome difficulties. This would be a tremendous advantage to me in the years ahead.

No matter where we lived, my parents ensured we always had a nurturing and stable home life. We went to church, prayed before meals, and spent time together as a family. They taught me how to pray and how important God was in my life. My childhood memories are happy ones, of our fun family movie and game nights, of our many camping trips, learning a deep love and appreciation for the outdoors, and of the intellectual stimulus of puzzles and faith-based studies we shared. I cherished this closeness and stability; it became an essential part of my life, a foundation that would prove crucial for my journey ahead.

I was a tiny, quiet, shy child who was not entirely comfortable in social situations. Instead, I found solace, relaxation, and renewal when I spent time exercising in the great outdoors. I discovered that I loved athletic activity, although because I was so tiny, I did not excel at nor participate in team sports. I channeled that love into long-distance running in middle school but did not compete. In high school, I participated and competed in cross-country running, cross-country skiing, and long-distance track. Through these sports, I learned discipline. I learned how to set goals for myself and achieve them. I learned how to persevere through difficulties. I learned how to endure present pain to benefit a future goal. And I learned that I loved being fit and healthy, a love I never abandoned.

My life after high school followed the usual pattern: I went to college and graduated with a degree in Chemistry, got married, and raised a family. God blessed me with two beautiful daughters, Nancy, and Kristy, whom I adored. I taught them my faith and love of God and how to care for others. They would one day become my fortress amid the storm.

My faith grew firm and unshakable, a sustaining bedrock for my life. I was not flamboyant about it, but it was rooted deep within my soul. I studied how to pray effectively and developed a close personal relationship with God. The hymns I learned and the scriptures I studied were a treasure trove of knowledge and inspiration; I often turned to them for guidance throughout my life. This faith was my lifeline; it supported and consoled me through the traumas of divorce and job loss and rejoiced with me in the blessings of my grandchildren. I cherished it deep within my heart; it was the single most important definition of who I was.

I continued my athletic endeavors and discovered a love for endurance bicycling, riding many miles over the years. I dedicated myself to exercise and a healthy lifestyle; I felt fit and happy and seldom got seriously sick. I was hospitalized only twice in all those years, once for toxic shock and once for appendicitis, and both times, I felt the Presence of God sustaining and healing me. I considered myself blessed that I was able to resume my healthy lifestyle quickly.

As I got older, my health continued to be strong; my doctors were amazed that I did not have to take the multitude of prescriptions that were deemed standard for most people my age to maintain their basic health. I attributed all that to good genes and my healthy athletic lifestyle. I was not prepared for what was to come.

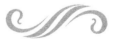

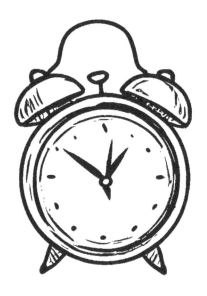

Symptoms and Realization

In early October, I was awakened from sleep in the middle of the night by a pain so intense that I had difficulty breathing.

In June 2022, I became marginally aware of some things in my body that were not normal for me, minor changes that individually seemed easily explainable. After all, I'd always been extremely healthy and athletic and had been making healthy changes to my diet in the previous several years. I was not worried—yet.

I had some tightness in my bladder, the kind you get just before you come down with a UTI. I had those before, so I trotted off to the store for cranberry juice and vitamin C, which I took regularly anyway and had been helpful on previous occasions. I knew that if I could head it off naturally, I would not have to get medical help, but if this didn't work, I would make an appointment with my doctor. The tightness came and went over the summer, and I thought I was successfully heading off the infection.

Around this time, I had to loosen my belt one notch. That may not seem concerning to most people, but in retrospect, it was an unaccustomed change for me. I had always had a completely self-regulating metabolism, and changes to my shape or weight were foreign to me. I mulled it over in my mind for days, wondering what it could mean. I reasoned with myself that I could just be getting older, as such changes were common for the population in general. I was over 60, after all; 62, to be precise. I had heard about weight gain being common after menopause, and surely that is what it was. I redoubled my exercises and closely monitored my intake.

In late August or early September, I began noticing a recurring feeling of being bloated, like when you have bad gas in your intestines. I had not changed my diet in any way I could correlate it with, so this was confusing. Again, I attributed this to the possibility of me just getting older and my body changing. It was not debilitating or painful and seemed to be intermittent, so I filed this away in the back of my mind with the other things and went on about my business. My birthday came and went; I was now 63.

Eventually, the bloating became undeniable and externally obvious. When I looked at my belly, it seemed poochy or swollen but without pain, tenderness, or firmness. Once again, I chalked it up to an age-related failure. I redoubled my efforts to tone the area, doing crunches, sit-ups, and isotonic exercises. The swelling seemed to come and go, and once again, I was convinced that I had identified and solved the issue.

As the summer wound down, and these trivial things continued to come and go, I began to reconsider my opinion that these separate minor changes were due to age or menopause. I had been menopausal at that time for about ten years. Changes related to the transition usually occur at that time and not years later. So, if not due to menopause, I wondered what could be causing these signs and symptoms.

In the back of my mind, quiet warning bells began to sound, and I started recalling discussions of certain women's problems that didn't manifest until they reached an advanced stage. I also reminded myself that any change to your body unaccustomed to your normal state should be examined further. By now, these symptoms had been persisting quietly for several months. I was beginning to think maybe there was something bigger going on here.

The swelling in my belly was growing more pronounced; I had begun taking pictures to document the changes. My belly button began to protrude, and it looked like I was pregnant. My mom didn't think it looked right, and we prayed for discernment and healing. I wondered again if I should call the doctor but inexplicably delayed in doing so.

In early October, I was awakened from sleep in the middle of the night by a pain so intense that I had difficulty breathing. It felt like extremely sharp gas pains. By the time I went to work, it had not subsided. I was having difficulty concentrating and bending over, and I began to make plans to notify my doctor. I sent him pictures of my latest belly expansion, along with a description of my symptoms. When the pain subsided later that day, I was still convinced that this was just gas, a belief I stubbornly clung to through the first set of doctor's visits even as my world shifted around me.

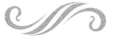

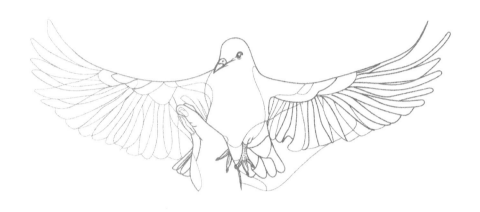

Doctors and Diagnosis

The doctor's response was short and direct:

this patient needs to be seen.

he doctor's response was short and direct: this patient needs to be seen. The office scheduled me for the very next morning. It was obvious that the doctor was concerned; the speed of the appointment spoke to that. I solaced myself by reasoning that since he had not sent me to the ER that very night, he obviously did not consider it an imminently life-threatening condition and was not gravely concerned. I would shortly come to understand just how uninformed I had been.

I love my primary care doctor. He is a kind and cheery man, and his demeanor with me has always been empathetic and efficient. I was comfortable that we had always agreed on my natural approach to my health. When he saw me that next morning, he asked me a long series of questions, but even when none of the conditions he was looking for seemed to apply to me, a caring smile remained on his face.

We looked at my distended belly, and he showed me how it responded to his probes. He diagnosed it as ascites, a condition in which the abdominal cavity abnormally retains fluid. Most of the time, on the first prognosis, this is related to liver failure. He seemed as perplexed as I was since I had no markers for any liver issues.

He ran a battery of blood tests, along with an X-ray and ultrasound, as well as scheduling me for a paracentesis to drain the excess abdominal fluid. I went home and googled ascites, which frightfully informed me that this stage of ascites and liver failure had an extremely poor prognosis. This was becoming very alarming.

When the lab and scan results came back the next day, the liver markers and X-ray were puzzlingly healthy, but the ultrasound had some shadowing in the pelvis and bladder, so he then referred me for a CT scan and to see a urologist. The scan was performed a few days later, and the results were sent to his office.

The following week, when I arrived at the hospital for my paracentesis, the swelling and fluid had decreased enough on their own that they were unable to perform the procedure. Once again, I reassured myself that this was a good sign and that surely all was well. The prayers seemed to be working.

When the doctor's office called with the CT scan results, everything suddenly changed. This scan was more defined and showed I had an adnexal mass. When I looked that up, it meant that I had an abnormal growth in the area around and between my left ovary and the fallopian tube. He canceled the urologist referral and referred me to a gynecological oncologist. He marked the referral as urgent.

I had a science background; I knew what that second word meant. I could not wrap my mind around the concept; the word 'cancer' whispered quietly in the back of my mind, but it felt utterly disorienting to me. I was still telling myself that we were continuing the search for answers, didn't have a definitive response, and that this referral was just for reassurance, but I was devastated.

I made a video call to my mom and dad that very night, and we cried and prayed together for quite some time. During our prayers, I felt an overwhelming sensation of peace, and I knew beyond the shadow of a doubt that I was in God's hands, that whatever happened and no matter how this turned out, He was in control and was taking care of me. Despite the whirlwinds of activity that were about to happen, that comfort and peace never once left me and guided and sustained me through it all.

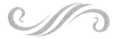

The Waiting

People traveled across the country to this world-class clinic,

and here I was, sitting on its very doorstep.

I was referred to Dr. Michael Gold at the Oklahoma Cancer Specialist and Research Institute in Tulsa, Oklahoma. I trusted my primary care doctor intimately and knew he had made the best professional choice for me, but I had no knowledge or experience in this area. Once again, I turned to my research, looking for information about this doctor and clinic. This facility was right here in my hometown! As I read about their credentials and reviews, I was amazed by the level of professional expertise and qualifications that I found. People traveled across the country to this world-class clinic, and here I was, sitting on its very doorstep. Once again, God had provisioned for me.

While I was waiting for the cancer clinic to schedule my initial appointment, I was instructed to go back to the clinic where I had the CT scan and pick up a copy of those results to take with me to that appointment. I requested and received two, so I would also have one to keep. It was quite interesting to navigate around my insides, looking at all the organs and bones.

A month went by without a call from the cancer clinic, and once again, I reassured myself. Surely, this was not really such a grave issue after all, or the response would have been more immediate, or so I thought.

At the beginning of November, I kept my previously scheduled annual physical appointment with my regular doctor. He was quite concerned that I had not yet been seen and repeated the call to the cancer clinic, again marking it urgent. Additionally, he referred me to a radiologist to see if we could get something moving sooner, and somewhere about this time, the cancer clinic called and scheduled my initial appointment with them for the Monday after Thanksgiving. The approaching storm clouds were gathering.

I had my secondary appointment with the radiologist just before Thanksgiving. My oldest daughter, Nancy, insisted on driving over from Norman to be with me on this visit. It was to be the first of many. I was nervous to see what they would find but comforted by my daughter's presence.

The radiologist looked at the scan on the disk I had brought and looked at my belly. She told me the mass was the size of a grapefruit, that it had probably been growing in there for quite some time, and that it needed to come out immediately, but this was different from her area of specialty. She told me that this kind of growth did not respond well to radiation and began looking for a referral in her network that had an immediate opening. Her first choice was unavailable, but she knew of and gave high marks to Dr. Gold and the clinic I was scheduled to see the next week, urging me to keep that appointment. I viewed this first outside appointment as my second opinion, and it helped validate and prepare me for what was to come.

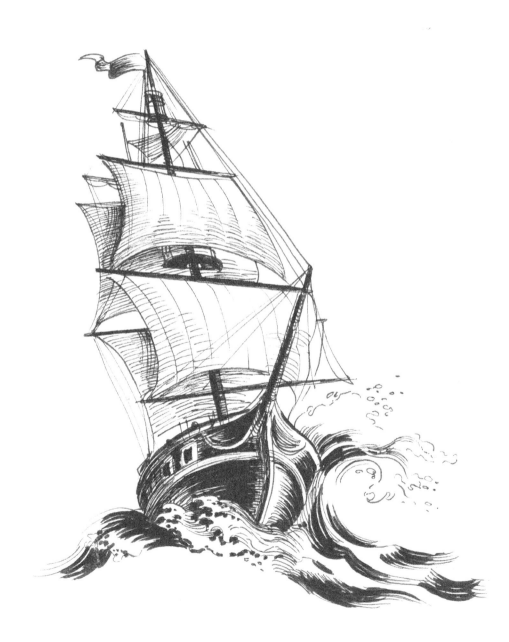

The Maelstrom

I was stunned and confused; I still had not entirely accepted the idea that this mass could actually be cancer, even though I was now sitting in a facility dedicated exclusively to the treatment and care of cancer patients.

On Monday, November 28, 2022, I walked into the cancer clinic, OCSRI, for the very first time. The facility was quite impressive—clean, bright, and modern, and the staff was kind and caring. In all the time I spent in this facility, I never met any one of them who did not exhibit this compassion and genuine concern for the people who came through their doors. I was confident that God had indeed brought me here.

My wonderful daughter Nancy was with me again, and I would come to rely on her as my primary caregiver in the months ahead. Her smile always brightened the room, and her excellent detailed notetaking assured us that we retained all the information from the whirlwind encounters. I believe that she had been specially prepared for this caregiver role, as she had recently dealt with both an extended illness and the death of a beloved pet and had supported a close friend in her cancer journey. Her knowledge and preparation were to be invaluable to me.

After the front desk, our first stop was the intake office, where we filled out paperwork, which included an optional Advanced Directive and Living Will/DNR. I was stunned and confused; I still had not entirely accepted the idea that this mass could actually be cancer, even though I was now sitting in a facility dedicated exclusively to the treatment and care of cancer patients. These were end-of-life documents; I felt fine; why was I being asked to fill them out now? I didn't know what all this meant for me yet, but I knew I wasn't ready to die, and it all seemed so final. Tears were becoming a big part of my life, and there were plenty of them that day. I would come to understand in the coming months that not all cancer patients have the options and outcomes that I was to experience.

The next stop was bloodwork. At that time, all medical facilities were still under pandemic restrictions, and my daughter had to wait in the hall while I went to get blood drawn. Then, we were sent upstairs to wait in the reception area for the call to the exam room. This routine was to become awfully familiar in the months ahead.

We were called, and the nurse took vitals while we waited for Dr. Gold, who would be my ally and advocate for the next several months. When he came in, he reviewed the notes and the disk of my previous CT scan with us. I immediately noticed his warm and caring eyes above the mask. This was no clinically dry expert. This man had immense compassion and a bedside manner that felt like a big, warm hug from your favorite uncle or like being wrapped in a soft, warm, fuzzy blanket. I liked him immediately.

The physical exam was quick and efficient, and once again, we heard the confirming news that this mass needed to come out. Sitting there with the sheet still over my knees, we listened to hear the options, but I was not prepared for him to lean forward then and ask with immense kindness and gentleness in his voice, "How does Thursday sound?"

I took a deep breath and a slight pause, and with tears in my eyes and a lump in my throat, I weakly nodded Yes. The room was spinning. This was suddenly happening so fast! But this man, with the demeanor of the angels, waited for me to regain my composure and gently confirmed that I was sure. Three times, he reverified that I was okay with my decision. I had only just met this man and already trusted him implicitly. The meeting with the radiologist the week before had prepared me for the outcome, so even though this timing was so unexpectedly sudden after all the waiting, I knew with absolute certainty that it was the right decision. The sooner we got this thing out of me, the better.

I was grateful for my daughter Nancy being there; her immaculate and detailed notes would be invaluable for recalling details and instructions when my brain was often overwhelmed with the avalanches of information. She wore a groove on the highway and often traveled to be with me for every appointment, and there were so many of them. She was my rock throughout this maelstrom of activity and perfectly placed in my hour of need. God brings us angels when we need them.

Things began to move extremely fast; a mere two days later, we were sitting in a room getting preoperative instructions, and the very next day, Thursday, December 1st, we were back for the big event. We were not the first surgery of the morning since we had been scheduled to fill an opening on such short notice. We waited, scared but glad to be there, nonetheless.

Once prepped and lying on the gurney, I requested the house chaplain for prayer. I had been reasonably calm up to this point. God and prayer had always been a big part of my life, and it seemed entirely appropriate to include Him now.

When the medic came to wheel me out of the room, however, I suddenly began to cry and reached out for a last touch from my loved ones there with me, Nancy, and Kevin. I knew that I was safe and well cared for, but the pent-up emotions and stress of the last week burst forth in wave after wave of tears and sobbing. Then I was whisked off down the hall, and they were left behind.

The staff parked me in a holding area while the operating room was prepped, and as I lay there alone in the dark waiting, I prayed. That same heavenly Peace enveloped me and calmed me, and I knew that my God was carefully watching over me.

When they wheeled me in, the operating room was very bright and cold. I was moved over from the gurney to the operating table and given layers of warm blankets as they hooked up all the machines, and then I was out. My loved ones, Nancy, and Kevin, waited in the reception area for the outcome.

The surgery went well but not entirely as planned. Dr. Gold performed a radical hysterectomy and debulking, which removed my ovaries, fallopian tubes, and connecting structures, the uterus, cervix, and omentum, the fatty layer that protects the abdominal organs. All of this, along with the primary tumor, was sent to pathology. In addition, he washed the peritoneal cavity to flush away any hidden malignant cells.

There was no evidence of any affected lymph nodes, which was a bright note. Still, there were multiple small, implanted growths scattered throughout my abdomen and intestines, which he patiently found and thoroughly excised. The largest of these, however, was growing on the outside of my lower colon to the extent that he had to call in a GI specialist to work on that area. Although this required considerable additional time, the GI surgeon could carefully scrape the lesion and remove this growth without additional complications.

The additional surgical work meant that I had now been in surgery much longer than expected, and my loved ones were growing concerned as the waiting room leaderboard continued showing no recent updates on my progress. Nancy was their primary coordinator and kept everyone grounded. Eventually, I was finished, and Dr. Gold reported to them that I had done great in surgery, that he had gotten everything he could find, and that he saw no residual disease.

The cancer was staged as grade 3C, High-Grade Serous Adenocarcinoma, with multiple secondary malignancies scattered throughout the peritoneum and peritoneal fluid. Where optimal results are defined as reducing the tumor to less than 1 cm, Dr. Gold defined mine as better than optimal, an optimistic prognosis from a cancer doctor. God had indeed put this man in my life and guided his hands. From that very moment, I was a cancer survivor.

After an overly lengthy stay in recovery, I was moved to my room. Nancy continued to drive over daily to visit and support me in the hospital, and she and Kevin took turns sitting with me, which I greatly appreciated. Once I was walking and off the pain pump, my abdominal drain was removed, and I was sent home on Monday, December 5th. It was frightful to look down and see those 47 staples marching up my belly where the swelling had been such a brief time before, but I tolerated them well.

We were to come back for post-surgical care in two weeks. If I thought this maelstrom of appointments and procedures had been a wild and bumpy ride so far, I was now about to experience the roller coaster ride of my life.

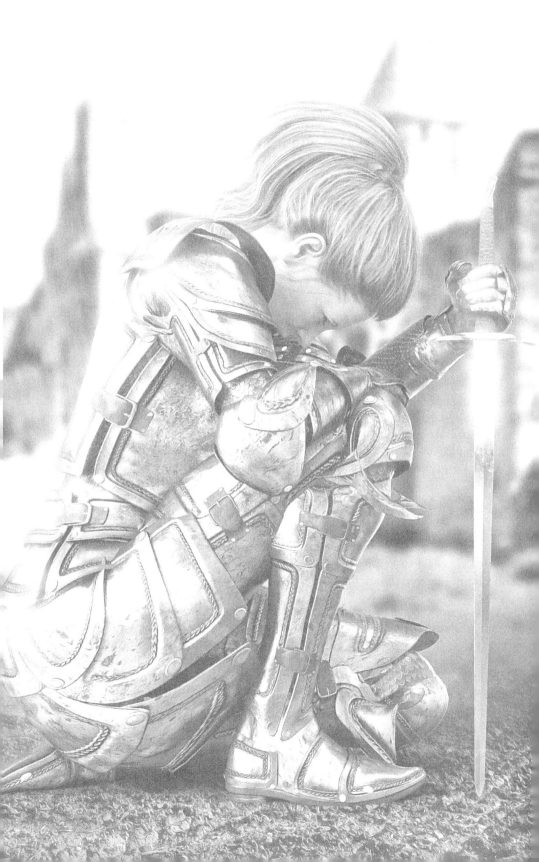

Chemo and Clinical Trial

My daily morning prayer time was becoming more focused and intimate.

I felt as if God was speaking to me directly.

The week before Christmas, I was back at the clinic to have my staples removed. We again followed the soon-to-be-familiar routine of getting bloodwork and then went upstairs to see the doctor. After the nurse removed my staples and replaced them with steri-strips, Dr. Gold's exam confirmed that I was healing nicely, and he gave me a work release. It may sound odd, but I was eager to get back to work. The activity and routine would feel familiar, and I missed my customers.

This meeting marked the beginning of my personal experience with chemotherapy. I had only a vague idea previously of what it entailed. My past impressions of it were colored by memories of friends I had seen become ghostly and frail from the powerful drugs, feebly living out their last days emaciated and in pain. I had once thought that if I were ever in such a position, I would refuse, yet here I was. Once confronted with the discussion, the decision was made and slipped almost unnoticed. I did not feel frightened but instead had a heavenly confidence that I had been led to this place and these people. The Peace of God continued to comfort and sustain me.

Dr. Gold presented us with a wealth of information, my options, and a chance at a clinical trial, which I eagerly accepted. His immediate goal for me was remission, with the ultimate treatment intent being curative, an ambitious target for a cancer doctor. My head was spinning from the volumes of information, and I was once again glad that Nancy was there with her superb note-taking skills.

The beginning of January 2023 was a bewildering flurry of appointments and procedures. There were more CT scans, more bloodwork, preliminary genetic screening, trial consultations, and the surgical placement of a central venous catheter, through which I would receive my infusions and would also be used for the multiple CT scans I would receive. I was incredibly grateful to have this port, as it would spare my thin veins from the trauma of repeated access and damage from the powerful drugs.

My daily morning prayer time was becoming more focused and intimate. I felt as if God was speaking to me directly. Each morning, He would bring a pertinent hymn or image to my mind, which would stay with me throughout the day. Friends and family around the world were praying for me, and I felt the confidence that their support provided me every day.

We attended an orientation class at the clinic, where I was given a blue book that would become my treatment Bible and my constant companion throughout my treatments. I learned about the potential for multiple side effects from the powerful chemotherapy drugs and which warning signs to watch for complications. I learned about blood counts, hydration, support groups, and hair loss, among others. This was becoming very real, and many tears were shed that day.

I would receive Carboplatin and Paclitaxel delivered in six rounds every three weeks from January through April, with a side serving of my clinical trial drug, Oregovomab. Since this stage three trial was a double-blind study, neither I nor my doctor would know if I received this drug or the placebo. Participating in this trial was important to me because it could benefit me and others who came after me.

The most surprising and difficult hurdle I encountered during this time was mentally wrestling with the upcoming hair loss. These drugs were a powerful poison and targeted fast-growing cells, damaging or killing not only the cancerous ones but non-discerningly any other such cells in the body, including hair follicles and bone marrow. At this time, I had beautiful, long, wavy, knee-length hair, which I was immensely proud of, but not in vain. I had long hair for my entire adult life, but it was not what defined who I was; I was a child of God, and that was what defined me. I was not afraid of losing it, or how I would look, so I was quite confused at the intensity of the emotions that I was experiencing. Wave after wave of tears occurred whenever I remembered the time was approaching. If it wasn't about the hair, what could it be? I kept searching for answers.

Nancy had a meeting during this time designed to give caregivers like her information about the myriad possible changes and challenges we both were about to encounter. She learned about a condition called dissociative grief, in which grief effects are felt in an area not directly related to the cause of the grief. This was my answer. The pattern of my emotional distress fit perfectly with the well-known stages of grief; this made it easier to understand and accept the emotions. The grief I was experiencing was not due to my hair loss but represented the change to my life as I had known it to that point, unplanned and irrevocable. Somehow, that made dealing with the impending loss easier to comprehend and tolerate.

The first round of treatment was scheduled for January 10th, with preliminary bloodwork and a doctor's exam on the 9th. This pattern was to be followed for each round of the series, with bloodwork and an exam the day before to verify that numbers were healthy enough for treatment. This first pair would be the baseline, and Nancy came over for both days as welcome support. We gathered all our supplies, enough to last the day since it would be long and full.

In my prayer time, the morning of my first treatment, I had a powerful vision. I was standing, and hanging in the air in front of me was a flaming sword, the Sword of the Spirit. In my vision, I grasped it firmly with both hands, slicing it back and forth in the air before me, defensively blocking and parrying. This was the Sword that struck down the flaming darts of doubt from the Evil One. It was a sign to me that God was quite literally there in the room with me, and we were ready to go together into battle with this demonic disease and beat it.

When Nancy arrived to take me to the clinic, I told her of my vision. She smiled quizzically and handed me a little gift bag. It contained an inspirational card and a T-shirt. On the front of this shirt was a woman clad in full armor, kneeling before the cross, and an inscription that read:

The devil whispered in my ear,

'You're not strong enough to withstand the storm.'

Today I whispered in the devil's ear,

'I have on the full armor of God.

I AM THE STORM!'

We looked at each other with tears in our eyes, amazed at the Lord's perfectly coordinated timing, acutely aware of God's presence with us as we set off for the clinic.

We arrived exceptionally early, the clinic's opening hours, so that we would have enough time for the long day ahead. We were ushered into a large, well-lit room with rows of cubicles containing treatment chairs. My wonderful nurses brought warm, heated blankets, which I loved, and accessed my port. Since I was a first-timer, they also brought me a bell to ring if I was in distress. We settled in, unsure of what the day would bring.

They first flushed my port and ran some saline solution; then, I received several bags of pre-meds of various kinds intended to combat the many side effects of the chemotherapy drugs. The heavy-duty Benadryl made me quite sleepy and loopy, but I was determined to stay awake and visit with my daughter, to hilarious effect.

The first bag of the chemo was Taxol and would take four hours to administer. It came to my cubicle in a biohazard bag, and the nurses donned scrub gowns, masks, and double gloves before opening it, reinforcing the gravity of the situation. The nurse started the drip, watched for a bit, and then returned to her station, reminding us of the bell and their nearby presence. We began putting on my cold therapy gloves and socks used to combat neuropathy; we jokingly referred to them as my Mickey Mouse gloves because they were so large and comically cumbersome.

Soon after this drip started, my stomach began to hurt just a little. I assumed it was nausea and asked for a nausea bag. Then, I also had a slight pain in my chest and leaned forward, moaning. Nancy grabbed the bell, but I assured her this was not an emergency. However, when the full anaphylactic reaction set in, it moved so fast I could not react. I could feel the curtain of unconsciousness rapidly closing in around me, and I tried to nod for the bell but could not speak. I collapsed forward and folded over onto my knees. Every inch of my skin had turned a vivid crimson red. This was now, in fact, a true emergency.

Nancy tried to ring the bell, but it was clenched too tightly in her hand and would not sound. The ever-vigilant nurses saw her distress, and every nurse on the entire floor responded to the emergency and came running to my aid. This reaction is common in first-time Taxol recipients, and they were ready. They stopped the Taxol drip, pushed some exceedingly strong recovery drugs, and monitored for recovery.

Even as I was collapsing, I felt no panic at all, just the Peace that had been with me since the night of that first phone call, and I also had confidence that the staff was well-trained and well-prepared. Although I was now unconscious, I could deliberately envision the same Sword from my morning vision. This time, I wielded it proactively and aggressively with a mighty grip, deliberately smiting and striking the spiritual shadowy forces.

As the recovery drugs took effect and I slowly regained consciousness, I began to see the nurses' feet and hear their voices. Once my muscles relaxed enough and I could sit up and speak coherently again, they restarted the drip without further incident. I finished the Taxol, the Carbo, and the clinical trial drug. It was an exceptionally long, exhausting day, and I was worn out. When the nurse asked if I wanted a wheelchair ride to the car, I gratefully accepted. There was a smile on my face; one down, only five more to go! I am convinced that God was with me that day; His presence was powerful.

I knew the time was approaching that my hair would begin to fall out. Typically, this is two weeks after this first treatment, and I ran out of time to decide what to do. It didn't seem logical to save it as a ponytail or make it into a wig, as there was no sentiment attached to the hair. I began to look at hair donation options. After researching several, I chose Wigs for Kids, an organization that provides wigs from donated hair to children with medical alopecia. I was pleased with this choice; it would bring good out of the chaos and joy to God's littlest angels. One of their registered stylists was in town, and I made the appointment.

The pattern of my after-treatment recovery was to become my standard experience for the days following each remaining treatment. I returned to work the very next day, feeling energetic and flushed from the steroids still circulating in my system. On day three, I would have some minor fatigue and headache that only lasted half the day and then receded. This would happen on Saturday, and I was completely ready to return to work on Monday. I was blessed to never have any more severe side effects than this during the whole time I was in treatment; I was acutely aware of the many prayers from people I knew around the world. Those prayers and my God sustained me throughout my entire cancer journey.

The week of my first treatment, I had my hair donation appointment on a Friday after work, and both of my daughters came with me for support. That morning, during my prayer time, I felt the distinct calling to dedicate this special gift to its intended purpose. I knelt on the floor in prayer and took my long hair out of its bun, laid it out across my upturned palms, and lifted it, dedicating my offering in prayer to God for His purpose and for His little ones. I felt an immense wave of joy as my offering was received. From that exact moment, though still attached to my head, it was no longer mine but His. I rose to my feet, put it reverently back up in the bun, and proudly carried this precious gift, now lovingly entrusted to my care, throughout the remainder of that day until the moment I would deliver it.

That evening, we met my stylist, Lexi, and shared my story with her. She was warm and compassionate and touched by our composure. I let down my long hair for the last time, and we prayed once more over the blessings it would provide the recipients. Lexi sat me in the chair and sectioned my hair into several ponytails, then used multiple zip ties down each one to keep the hair from tangling on its transit to the preparation facility.

The big moment- the first cut! There were many tears, of course, but they were tears of joy this time. This gift would be used for so much good. The rest were also removed from my head and placed on my lap. She finished with a cute pixie cut that would last me briefly before I lost the rest; then, we measured the donation and took pictures. I was able to donate 37 inches to this beautiful cause. It was a very emotional but satisfying evening.

I began documenting my transition with daily photos of my hair. Right on schedule, on day 14, I started noticeably thinning and experiencing scalp pain, and by day 16, it was coming out in clumps. I was prepared for this and used the shower as my catch basin. I combed my fingers through the curls and rinsed off the loosened globs of hair until no more came out. I had to clean the drain catcher multiple times before I was done. For such short hair, it seemed like a huge pile. This was the day of the most loss, though the thinning of what little was left continued throughout my treatments.

This was no longer an emotional process for me since it was now merely another side effect of my chemo. I took some silly photos when it resembled a Mohawk or the classic old man bald on top look; it tinged the transition with humor. There was now no longer any doubt that I was a cancer patient.

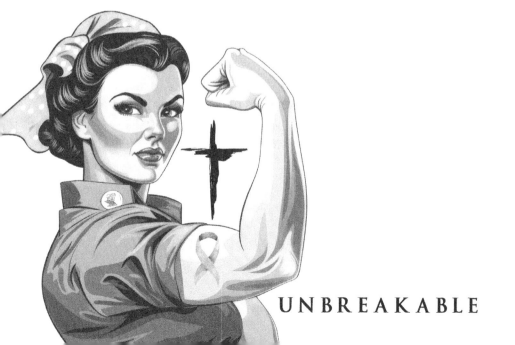

UNBREAKABLE

The Continuation

I passionately believed that God was the biggest reason

for my healing thus far; how could I not continue to trust Him?

eal is the ribbon color for ovarian cancer awareness, and as I needed a creative outlet for my pent-up energies, I began making jewelry and beanies in that color. The beanies would be helpful for hair replacement warmth, and the jewelry would become a visible sign of my invisible disease. I made many pieces for myself and my family throughout this time. The process was therapeutic and gave me a sense of positivity. Dr. Gold always noticed and appreciated each new piece. I found and customized a couple of teal ball caps; on one, I placed a cross dead center and the cancer ribbon emblem off to the side as a representation of my conviction that God was in charge and not cancer.

I returned to the clinic for rounds two and three, and the familiar routine made me feel more confident. The day prior, I was downstairs for bloodwork and upstairs for the office visit. Once my hematology blood counts were deemed acceptable, I was cleared for treatment the following day. My blood tumor marker count was responding exceptionally well to the treatments. This marker, CA-125, measures inflammation in the bloodstream caused by this cancer. While the marker by itself is not helpful as a reliable guide for diagnosis or a definitive absolute scale like A1C or other well-known blood markers, trends are important, and mine had fallen from 377 before surgery to 16 afterward, back into the normal range. By the second treatment, mine had fallen to below 1, marked undetectable, and my chart now proudly announced that I was NED, with No Evidence of Disease. This was big news! I credit God and the prayer support of all my prayer warriors, Dr. Gold, and the clinic staff for such outstanding results. Treatment three was then completed; I was halfway there!

Nancy was now coming over only on the days of treatment. She always brought a big smile and was my emotional and physical support caregiver through all the remaining treatments, helping me eat and drink. At the same time, I was too clumsy in my Mickey Mouse gloves and helping with the multiple cords and lines when I needed to go to the bathroom, which was often with all the additional fluids. We shared some extended mother-daughter time that I cherished even more since we didn't live in the same town, and visits were sometimes infrequent.

It was time for treatment four, and I was actively looking forward now to ticking each one off and reaching the end. I was tolerating the chemo exceptionally well, gaining rather than losing weight, and my color and energy were exemplary. It would have been difficult to tell I was a cancer patient if not for the hair loss and jewelry.

I arrived at the clinic in high spirits. I got my bloodwork and went upstairs to see the doctor. I was not prepared for his words. My neutrophil count, a white blood cell variant impacted by the powerful chemo drugs, was just barely too low for treatment, and he would not clear me. At first, I thought I could convince him to 'squeak me by,' but his tone was compassionately firm. He offered to redraw my blood in the morning to see if I passed, but if it didn't, I would have to wait another week for treatment. I was stunned and confused; was there anything I could do? The nurse and doctor exchanged glances; they had no answers. Finally, the nurse said I could climb stairs, but I could tell she was grasping at straws and offering platitudes.

I left the clinic feeling deflated and defeated. I discussed with Nancy whether to have her come over in the morning, with the very real chance of being turned away and having to come back only one week later. We decided to take the chance to pass the redraw and made plans for her to come. My spirits were reviving, and with an iron will, I took firm action. My work is a two-story warehouse, so I had stairs ready; I climbed them that day in multiple sets of reps until my legs were tired, and it was time to go home. I found a medical research paper online that explored the ability of extra dark chocolate to raise neutrophil levels, and I stopped for some on the way home; it couldn't hurt. I reminded myself that these protections were in place for my health and determined to accept gratefully whatever the outcome of the next morning would be. I called my mom and dad again for prayers and found stability and Peace in them. I spent the rest of the evening at home preparing by walking and eating my chocolate.

Nancy arrived early the following day, and we proceeded to the clinic. However, this time, we detoured to the lab for the blood redraw, then went upstairs and waited pensively while they were processed. We talked and prayed for me and the other patients waiting with us.

When the nurse showed up with my results, she had a huge grin on her face; I had passed, and not just by a little bit! Waves of elation and gratefulness swept over me, and of course, I was crying again; how was it possible that I was so happy in this place? We swept into the treatment room, elated to be proceeding. We settled in for the familiar routine, chatting and passing the time until the nurses withdrew access from my port, and we were free to go. Two-thirds done, and only two more rounds to go!

This week's appointments included a new CT scan, and I was elated that it continued to show no evidence of recurrent malignancy. I had now also had expanded genetic testing; when the results came back, they showed I did not have the mutations in my BRCA genes, which can mean an increased risk for breast or ovarian cancer. This was welcome news for me; it also meant I did not pass on those mutations and increased risk to my children. My CA-125 continued to remain undetectable. All these results were my proof that God was indeed taking care of me.

My Cancer Journey and the Faith that Sustained Me.

At my office visit for round five, Dr. Gold discussed an option available to me based on my genetic testing results for going on Parp inhibitors after I was done with my treatments. This class of drugs can enhance the effectiveness of chemotherapy and prolong the length of time it takes to remain disease-free. However, if I chose this pathway, I would not be able to stay in the clinical trial, which studied the long-term effects of its therapy unaided. There were also additional potential side effects to consider. This was a lot to think about; I requested additional time.

Nancy came for our fifth session, and we settled into the familiar routine. I discussed with her what the doctor had told me, and we discussed my options and thoughts. First and foremost, I did not want to leave the trial; it could still benefit both me and the trial results so that I could stay. I had not chosen to participate to drop out; I intended to see it through. Second, I had been blessed to have very minimal side effects throughout my treatments and was not too enthusiastic about the new chances for them here.

Last but not least, I passionately believed that God was the biggest reason for my healing thus far; how could I not continue to trust Him? Dr. Gold had told me that this decision was not irrevocable; I could begin the inhibitors at any time if we determined I needed them in the future. As Nancy and I discussed and weighed the information, our consensus fell in line with my initial inclination; I would choose to stay in the trial and decline the inhibitors. Packing up at the end of the day, I felt the familiar Peace of God confirming my decision. As we left the clinic, my excitement was palpable; I was five down, and there was only one more to go!

Dr. Gold had a teal cancer ribbon tattoo on his left forearm; when I asked about it, he told me he got it to represent his patients and his commitment to their healing. He also told me he was getting a starfish on the other arm, the staff's spirit animal. I was puzzled until I remembered the story of the older man tossing starfish back into the sea, who, when asked why he persisted when there were so many he could not save, replied that it had made a difference to the one he had just saved. It seemed an entirely appropriate metaphor for these people who saved lives.

I received excellent care and compassion from everyone at the clinic; they gave me exemplary care. I wanted to do something to thank them and turned to my crafts again. I found a beautiful blown glass starfish paperweight for Dr. Gold with teal swirls. I found keychains for my nurses with a tag that read, "Never underestimate the difference you made and the lives you touched." I added a starfish charm and a cancer ribbon charm to each, along with a small teal braid representing my ovarian cancer. The nurses also got angel pins, and I wrote a note of heartfelt thanks to Dr. Gold on a card, thanking him for making a difference in this starfish's life.

Round six was upon me; the finish line was in sight! I wore a violently teal wig and a gigantic smile to my exam. Everyone on the staff was surprised to see me in that wig but excited for me and impressed with my enthusiasm. I presented Dr. Gold with my card and gift, and he read my note with tears in his eyes and then gave me a big hug. It was a perfect token of my gratitude for the wonders he had performed for me. We agreed together that God had used him and guided his hands in my healing.

My red blood cell counts were a little low, but not enough to prevent treatment, so we were ready for the sixth and final round of chemo on April 27, 2023. Nancy wore a shirt that proudly proclaimed, "I wear teal for my Mom," and I wore one that said, "Ovarian Cancer Warrior—Unbreakable," with a depiction of a Rosie the Riveter-style woman wearing a teal cancer ribbon tattoo on her flexed bicep. I felt powerful wearing this message and my teal wig.

When we got to our station and settled in, my beautiful, creative, supportive daughter surprised me by pulling out multiple inspirational signs and banners she had found and printed, covering the walls of my booth with them. I sat surrounded by messages of hope: "I can't keep calm; today is my last chemo." "She wears her scars like a Warrior, reminding her she's Alive." "My God is stronger than ovarian cancer." These and so many more brightened our station and blessed my heart. She gave me a sweet card and a teal ceramic women's empowerment goddess mug, which I adored. I could not have asked for or found a more suitable caregiver.

The nurses brought me a Purple Heart Award certificate of completion, signed by all the staff members, which was a touching gesture. This was turning into quite the completion party. I presented my special nurses with their little tokens, and we took pictures. I had come to love these people with their cheery smiles and efficient demeanor. They told me to be sure to ring the bell on my way out, and Nancy and I discussed this option throughout the day. The time passed more quickly than normal due to my anticipation of completing my last treatment. Then, it was time to pack up, and we headed downstairs to ring the bell.

The bell at my clinic was located downstairs, away from the treatment rooms, and included a full wall labeled The Ribbon of Hope. It included inspirational sayings and a metal ribbon-shaped framework where past patients had hung pieces of ribbon with their own messages of support to future patients. We had not prepared for a bell ceremony; it seemed somewhat awkward and contrived, but after a full day of consideration and changes of heart, I decided to go ahead.

The hallway seemed deserted; we were there by ourselves. I had Nancy video me, a small unprepared speech, and a reading of the poem posted by the bell. I felt awkward and self-conscious but proceeded. But when the notes of the bell pealed out, there was an eruption of cheering. Every staff member in hearing, from the front desk personnel to the nurses passing by in the halls, stopped what they were doing and stood up, stepping into the aisles, clapping, and cheering for me. It brought tears of joy to my eyes, and I no longer felt alone. I raised my hands in the air in a victory salute of acknowledgment. My favorite part of the video is hearing Nancy cheering and whooping at the end.

Round six was completed; I was done! Looking back, this incredible journey seemed so short. All that had happened in the past few months condensed into swirling memories, overlaid with the Peace that had never left me and the Faith that had sustained me.

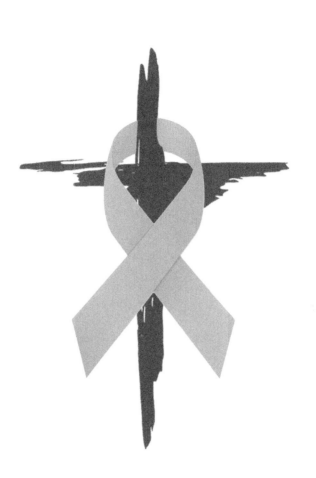

God's Promise
and My Commission

This crazy journey had been one of faith from the very beginning.

My treatment was over, but my journey was not. I began feeling a firm spiritual urging to tell of my faith and my resultant healing whenever and wherever the subject of my cancer journey was discussed. Since I was now virtually bald, this provided many such opportunities. I was not accustomed at that time to speaking with strangers about my faith but was firmly determined to obey the leading I was feeling. Throughout this journey, I was surrounded and supported by the prayers and faith of many people, family around the country, and friends old and new around the world. It was uplifting to see the responses and the confirmations of faith coming back to me in many of these discussions. These encounters strengthened my own faith and my relationship with God.

These encounters came in many forms, from discussions with friends or work companions to prayers from acquaintances of friends who had never met online friends, even from complete strangers. While visiting a favorite craft center, I met two sweet ladies one day. Upon discussing my cancer cap and telling the story of my cancer faith journey, they asked me to pray for them. Of course, I agreed. Once again, I felt that familiar Peace of God wash over and through me, and this prayer warrior told me that God had completely healed me from this cancer. Of course, I already knew that, but it was a sweet confirmation. I believe there are no chance encounters when God arranges the details; my father used to say there were no coincidences but called them holy-instances. For me, this unplanned meeting strengthened my faith and resolve to share my journey's story.

My morning prayer time continued to bolster me for each new day. I had the distinct impression that God was leading me to something bigger in telling my story, but the details were still unknown. The urge was increasing, but I would have to be patient and trust He would show me the plan in His time.

I had not seen my parents in person since this whole thing started. Still, they were traveling again after COVID-19 isolation, coming from far away Washington state to visit over Memorial Day weekend, and my sister came with them from Colorado. We had a wonderful visit, reconnecting after so much time apart. We hiked on local trails, and my forestry sister was excited to add new plant species to her watch list.

My lovely daughters planned a party for my chemo completion to share the joy together. Nancy made cakes and decorated them with teal cancer ribbons. I was surprised and delighted when I saw the decorations, which were all the same posters from that last day of treatment and my Purple Heart Award, brought back out and displayed. She changed the prominent poster to read, "I can't keep calm; I've finished my last chemo." She found a pack of small wedding bells, decorating them with teal; there were enough for each of us. I got inspirational cards from each of them and reread the bell poem. We all rang our bells together and cheered. My cherished family surrounded me this time, and it felt like a true celebration.

These family members had been the backbone of my prayer support team, and I wanted to show my appreciation for each of them, so I gathered my craft supplies once again. I made more bracelets and put together small appreciation packs for each of them. After more tears and hugs, I gave a synopsis of all I had been through and how much it meant to me that they had all been such a vital part of my journey and my healing, especially my mother, who had been a fervent prayer warrior from the very beginning, and my second daughter Kristy, who had given emotional support to Nancy when she was overly stressed from her caretaker role. I was glad that each of them was part of my support team and that we had such a strong family of faith warriors.

I was equally touched by their words of affirmation back to me. My sister told me that my faith humbled her. My father, whose strong example had shown me how to live a life of faith and taught me how to pray, thanked me for sharing my strong statement of faith. It was a powerful and emotional evening, and we celebrated with a delightful dinner. I was touched to see my father pull Nancy aside and express his personal appreciation for her faith and support. My heart was full.

I had one more treatment coming at the clinic, but this time, it was only for the clinical trial, the final dose. This was my opportunity to hang a ribbon on the Wall of Hope. I determined to find an appropriate message to write on my ribbon. I had been collecting inspirational quotes and awareness memes, but though I went back through all of them, none was the right one. I went to the fabric store and found the perfect ribbon, teal for OC and big enough for my message—one step at a time.

This crazy journey had been one of faith from the very beginning, not knowing what lay around each upcoming corner but trusting that I would be given the strength and wisdom for each challenge as it came. And so, it was with my ribbon. The week before I was due at the clinic, I found my message, spoken by God to Joshua as He prepared him for the challenges ahead and the calling on his life:

"Be strong and courageous. Do not be terrified.

Do not be discouraged.

For the Lord your God will be with you wherever you go."

Joshua 1:9

It was uplifting and perfectly appropriate. I printed it out and hung it on my bathroom mirror, where it continues to inspire me daily. I then inscribed it on my teal ribbon and initialed the reverse. Its consecrated message would bring hope to those who came after me.

When I went to the clinic, I wore the ribbon around my neck as a stole. Dr. Gold noted with appreciation the message inscribed upon it. He also noted that, while it was never a suitable time to get cancer, there was now a national shortage of Carbo, one of the primary chemo drugs, and I had finished before that happened. The timing was providential. Once again, I was blessed and grateful.

Nancy came over for treatment day, as she had since the very beginning. As we sat in the reception area waiting to be called, my research nurse came and sat and talked with us. We reminisced together and celebrated how well my treatments had gone and how blessed I was with my healing and NED status. At this point, as I gazed around the waiting room at the other patients, I felt overwhelmingly intense waves of compassion and grief wash over me again and again. These other patients were the ones who had not experienced the same excellent results that I had, and my heart ached for them. I spoke with Nancy and my nurse about how fervently I wished that every single one of these others could similarly experience the beneficial results I had. I began to cry softly at first, but with increasing intensity until I was sobbing. I felt enormous waves of God's love reaching out to each of them through me; they were so intense that they seemed like swirling bands of color washing the room in Peace and Hope. I continue to yearn and pray for the day that researchers find more advanced and effective treatments and cures for this beast we call cancer so that one day, all can be healed.

The treatment day this time was shorter than normal since I didn't have the full chemo drug dosages, and quite soon, it was time to go. The nurse brought me a wheelchair to ride downstairs, and we stopped in the hall by the Ribbon of Hope. I found a suitable spot on the wall, and we hung and tied my ribbon message, praying over it a dedication prayer. It was a holy moment.

My hair was now growing back. When the first growth came in, it was at first tiny, short, silvery golden halo fuzz, then became long enough to look intentionally short, and I abandoned my hats and wigs. It was the softest hair I'd ever had, as soft as a baby duck's downy butt; I couldn't stop touching it. It reminded me of the extra soft hair on a newborn's head that you keep rubbing with your nose. As it grew a little more, it reminded me of velvet, with a distinct nap. Eventually, the curls started showing. Each new stage was a fresh celebration of life. The renewal of my hair growth mirrored the renewal of my health, renewed growth, and a renewed outlook for the future.

Conjunctive with the growth of my hair was an increasing imperative to tell my story of how God was the central character in this drama, not the cancer. This imperative was so strong that I began calling it my commission, a virtual contract between me and my God who had saved me. I did not know yet what form this work would take, but I was confident that it would be revealed to me in His time.

At the end of July, I had my final exit appointment for the clinical trial. This included the same questionnaire that I had filled out when I started the trial, a physical exam, and a CT scan. The trial after-care meant that I would receive these extra exams at every follow-up, a bonus for me in confirming that no cancer returned. I was now well and truly done with my treatment phase; all that remained now would be follow-ups over the coming years and an appointment schedule going all the way out to 2027. My next appointment would be in October! It seemed surreal somehow, but with God in my heart, I danced out the doors of this place that had been a home of sorts for these past many months.

I still needed a clear directive on the form or method of my commission. I continued my morning prayer times; they had become an integral part of my day, and I waited for the next reveal. One night, I was awakened in the wee hours by a Holy Presence, imprinting a swirling word collage in my mind. The content was quite specific and complete, and I rehearsed it to myself for memorization, but I decided instead to write it down for the morning and go back to sleep. I had intended to rehash and rewrite the passage in the morning with a clear mind, but when I reviewed the message, it was apparent that it had been inspired and given complete. This was to be the opening of my story.

This small start was all that was given to me for weeks, and I continued to pray and wait expectantly for inspiration. The story flowed out of me when it came, and it settled on the pages almost effortlessly. I knew God was guiding my words. As I continued pouring out my heart, I relived each moment anew. The overarching theme was the promise of healing and of my faith. The cancer was no longer center stage.

This story is only the beginning; God has much for me yet to do. My faith and God's peace carried me through my journey with cancer. It is my fervent prayer that these words and this story will bolster your own faith and lead you to a deeper communion with God, Your Maker. He lives today and will be your Lord if you will but ask and listen.

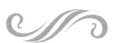

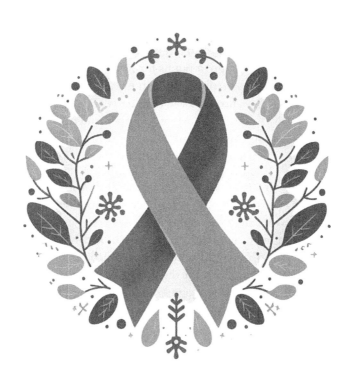

Afterword

Awareness

One thrust of my commission is to raise awareness of this dangerous gynecological cancer: not all cancer is pink. Early detection is critical; survivability is much greater before the malignant cells spread. Like shards of broken glass or sugar granules tossed into the wind, once scattered, it isn't easy to locate every single one.

Here, then, are some Ovarian Cancer awareness facts:

There are over 20,000 new cases of Ovarian Cancer worldwide each year, one every six minutes, and over 14,000 deaths.

It is the 17th most diagnosed cancer and the 5th deadliest cancer among women.

All women of any age are at risk for some form of gynecological cancer; 1 in 73 women will be diagnosed with OC in their lifetime.

Any person born with ovaries can develop OC.

A person can develop OC even after ovarian removal.

Only 20% of cases are found in the early stages; 60% or more of cases are diagnosed after metastasis.

Many cases are only found coincidently while researching other complaints.

Increased risk factors can include:

☐ A family history of breast or gynecological cancers.

☐ Mutations in the BRCA genes.

☐ Increasing age.

☐ Obesity.

☐ Hormone replacement therapy.

Factors that can decrease your risk include pregnancy, childbirth, breastfeeding, taking oral contraceptives, and a healthy diet and weight.

There is currently no medically accurate tool available for the early detection of OC- Pap smears do not detect OC.

Diagnostic tests can include CA-125 blood tests, pelvic exams and biopsies, CT or PET scans, X-rays, and transvaginal ultrasounds,

Listen carefully, ovarian cancer whispers. These early-stage symptoms are subtle and may not have any noticeable symptoms; many are signs of other conditions, making them easy to ignore or confuse with other common conditions. If you have any of these symptoms that persist for over two weeks, seek medical advice.

Bloating- a persistent feeling of being bloated or having gas, abdominal swelling

Early satiety- consistently not being able to eat as much, feeling full quickly, indigestion

Abdominal pain- persistent abdominal, pelvic, and lower back pain or cramps

Changes in bowel or bladder habits- frequent urge to urinate or changes in bowel habits, constipation

Heightened fatigue- constant fatigue, especially combined with these other symptoms, that interferes with your daily lifestyle, shortness of breath

Weight change- gain or loss without changes to diet or exercise

Concern that this is not normal for you- listen to your body

Make sure you and your loved ones know these signs and symptoms and pay attention to your body. If it feels wrong, keep speaking up until your voice is heard. I had many of these very subtle signs, but I am an ovarian cancer survivor today because I eventually listened and acted.

Cancer is not a death sentence; advances are being made in this field daily. If you do require treatment, make sure you seek out a qualified gynecological oncologist rather than just a regular oncologist or gynecologist. The knowledge and skill of this type of specialist crucially improve the outcome of treatment for this cancer; results are up to five times more positive.

Do not be afraid to be your own advocate. The decisions you make may save your life.

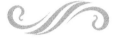

FIGHT LIKE A girl!

Resources

- National Ovarian Cancer Coalition
  https://ovarian.org
  888-OVARIAN (888-682-7426)
  214-273-4200
  nocc@ovarian.org

- Ovarian Cancer Research Alliance
  https://orcahope.org
  866-399-6262
  212-268-1002

- Oklahoma Cancer Specialist and Research Institute
  https://ocsri.org
  800-556-6056
  918-505-3200

- Tenaciously Teal
  https://www.tteal.org/
  405-753-4496
  tenaciouslyteal@gmail.com

- Harts of Teal
  https://hartsofteal.org

- Ovarcome
  https://ovarcome.org
  713-800-2976
  info@ovarcome.org

- National Cancer Institute
  https://www.cancer.gov
  800-422-6237
  NCIinfo@nih.gov

- American Cancer Society
  http://cancer.org
  800-227-2345

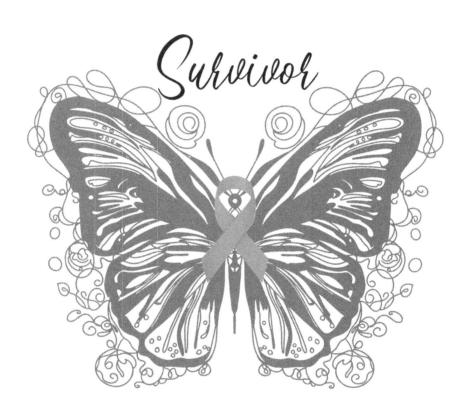

Epilogue

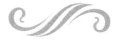

I had my second follow-up in January 2024, a CT scan on Monday, and a doctor's visit on Wednesday. As always, I was expecting great news and great results. I had no fears because the God who loves me continued to infuse and saturate me with the Peace That Passes Understanding.

I have never experienced what cancer patients like to call "scanxiety", the feeling of dread that comes before a procedure that will tell if the cancer has returned, or afterwards when waiting for the results of those tests to be made known. I went to the clinic and had my scan in good spirits but did not expect to know the results until my doctor's visit two days later.

On Tuesday, I saw that the results had been posted in my patient portal, and I was eager to open and view them on my computer, when the strangest thing happened. I felt an intense sensation of dread and hesitation. I put my hand down and paused. I tried again, and once more for a third time, with the same results. Then, I realized this was an attack of doubt from the enemy! I stood up, walked away from the computer, put on my prayer clothes, and communed with God for a time. He restored my Peace, and we wrestled with and banished the Deceiver. "I know who you are, and you don't belong here. I am a child of God! GET OUT!!!!!"

Only then did I go back and open the portal. I knew that I remained healed by God's grace, and the scan results confirmed that I was clear of recurrent or metastatic malignancy. The devil knows where to hit and produce doubts, but my faith in God drove out the fear.

In early 2024, I was selected as one of the fashion show runway models for Care Packs and Cocktails, sponsored annually by Tenaciously Teal, an ovarian cancer advocacy organization based in Oklahoma City. It was a great honor and the start of my journey through the after-cancer advocacy life. Continuing to do events like this will inspire others and give them hope as they find their way through this overwhelming change in their lives.

I am a fighter, a survivor, a woman of faith and strength- I am a "surthrivor". I continue to remain NED and clear of cancer; I owe it all to God and His healing presence in my life. I am and always will be completely His.

Photo Memories

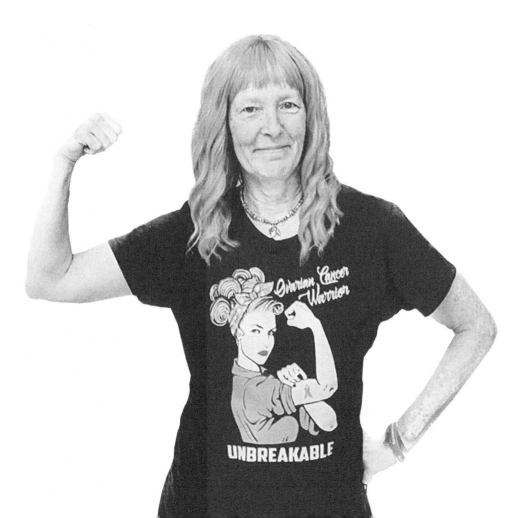

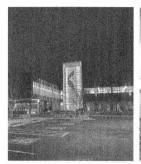

The clinic that would be
my chemo home (OCSRI)

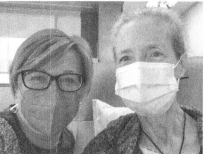

Nancy and I

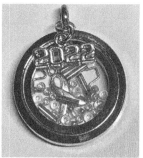

The locket I made from
my surgery staples

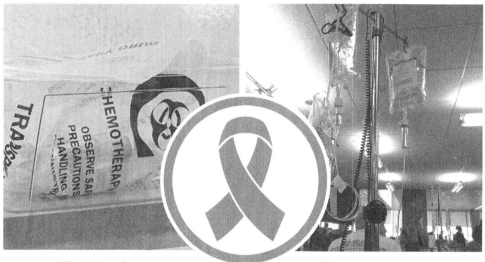

Toxic chemo bag

My view of the chemo pole

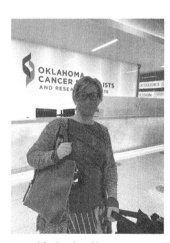

My daughter Nancy on our
first day of chemo

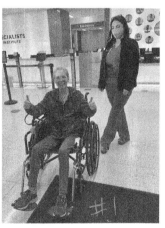

Success! One down, five to go!

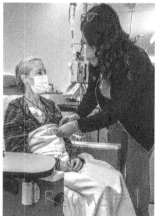

Hooking me up for Round #1

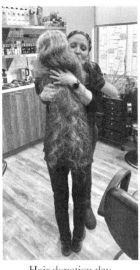

Hair donation day

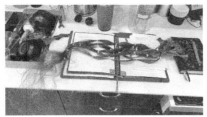

My donation to Wigs For Kids

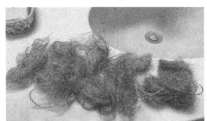

The hair as it came out

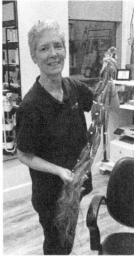

37" of blessings for God's little angels

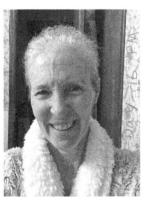

Losing the hair

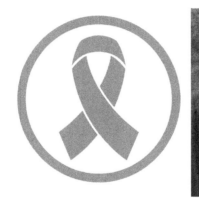

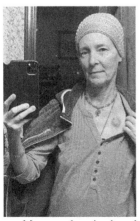

The full armor of God

My port and repping the teal

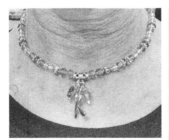

Cancer jewelry

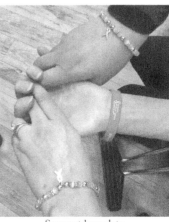

Support bracelets

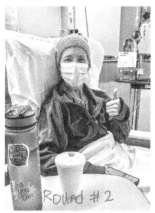

Round #2- No turning back

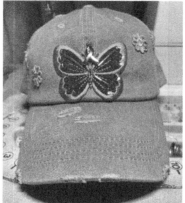

The teal hat I customised

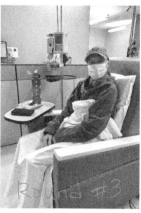

Round #3 and halfway done!

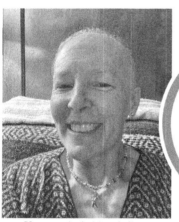

Happy to be bald and alive

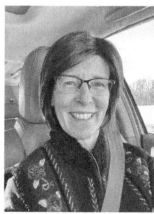

Looking like a little old man

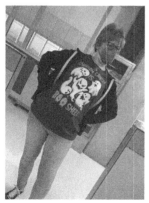

My daughter had the BEST shirts!

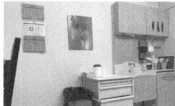

Exam room

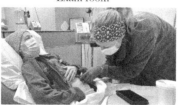

Administering pre-meds

My favorite red wig

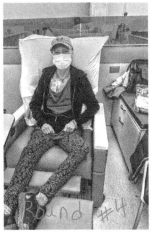

Round #4- two thirds
done and going strong

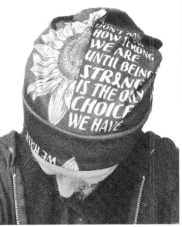

We don't know how strong we are until
being strong is the only choice we have

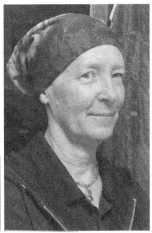

Beanie style

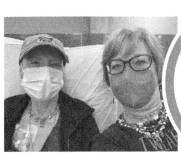

Me and Nancy

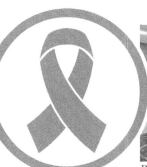

Round #5 and only one more to go!

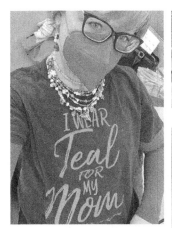

My best support caregiver

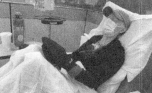

Resting with the cold gloves

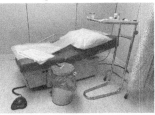

The 'favorite' couch

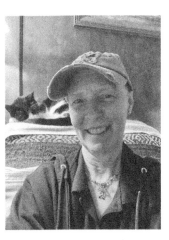

God is my faithful companion

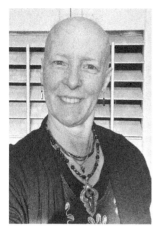

God is alive and my
constant companion

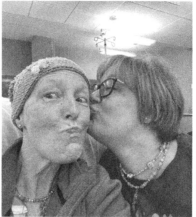

Round #5 and only one more to go!

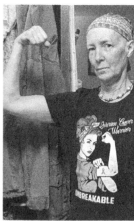

Unbreakable!

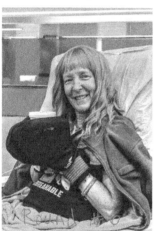

My "Mickey Mouse" gloves

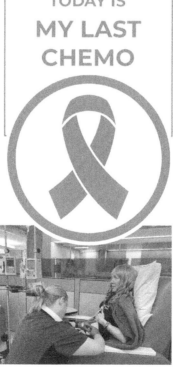

I CAN'T KEEP CALM
TODAY IS
MY LAST CHEMO

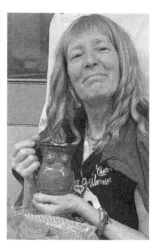

Women's empowerment mug

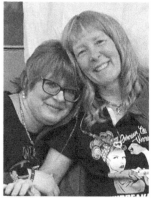

Last time for the cold gloves and socks

More pre-meds

Nancy and I

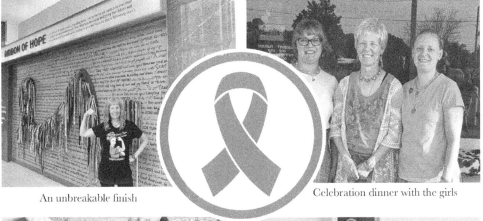

An unbreakable finish

Celebration dinner with the girls

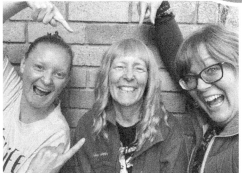

Me and the girls celebrating

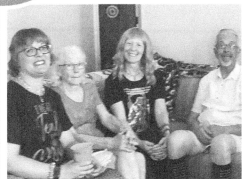

My family

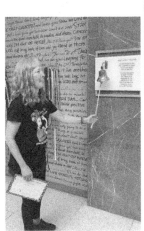

Ringing the bell!

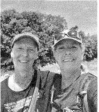

Me and my sister

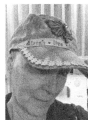

The cross banishes the cancer!

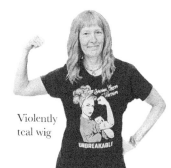

Violently teal wig

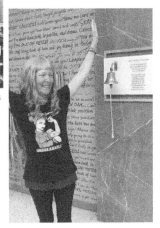

Celebration of completion

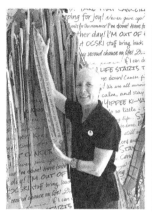
Praying my message for
those who come after

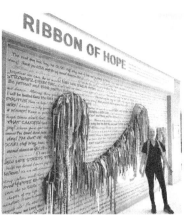
Ribbon of Hope

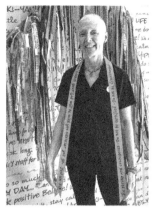
The Lord your God will be
with you wherever you go

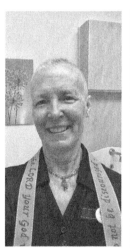
Teal's the deal

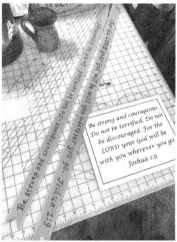
Joshua 1:9 for my ribbon of hope

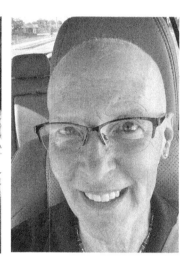
Look! new hair!

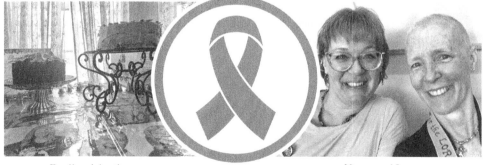
Family celebration   Nancy and I

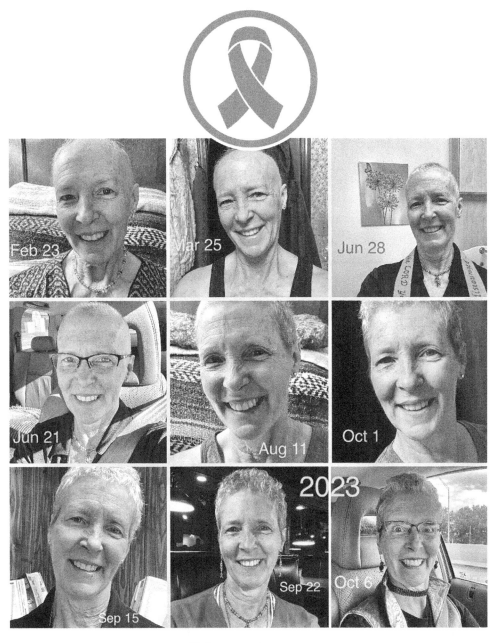

Hair regrowth progress

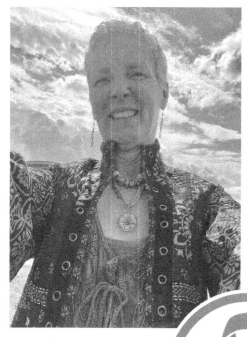

Happy birthday to me!

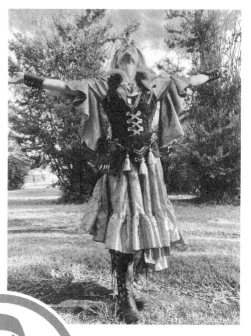

Teal Warrior celebrating life!

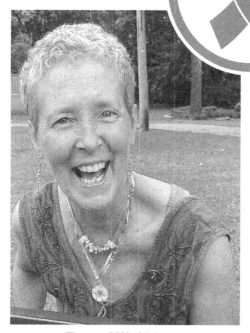

The pure JOY of living!

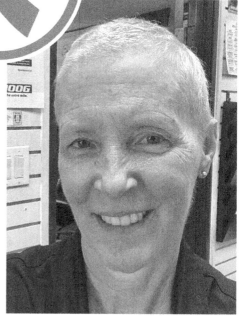

Soft bunny hair

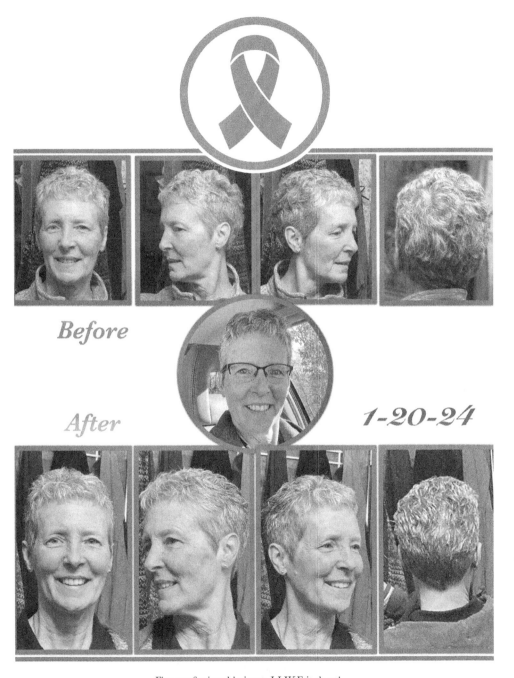

Before

After

1-20-24

First professional haircut- I LIKE it short!

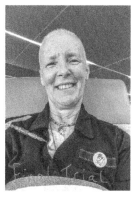

Final time in the chair

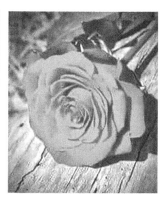

National Ovarian
Cancer Coalition

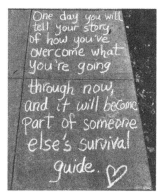

Overcoming

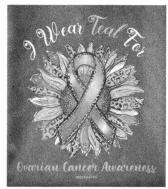

Ovarian Cancer Awareness https://
www.facebook.com/ovariancancer
awarenesss?mibextid=LQQJ4d

Teal for Ovarian cancer

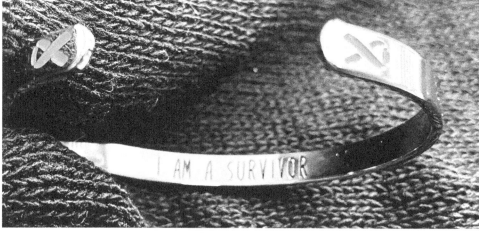

I am a survivor

Introducing the Class of 2024
Care Packs & Cocktails
Models

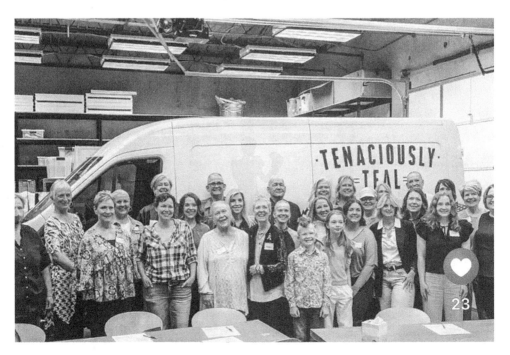

Care Packs and Cocktails

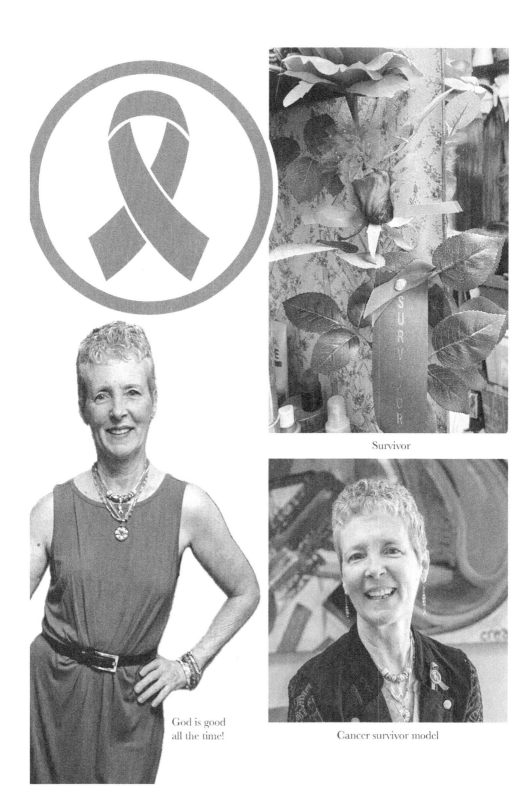

Survivor

God is good
all the time!

Cancer survivor model

Made in the USA
Coppell, TX
26 September 2024

37772428R00052